# Alzheimer's/Dementia
## from the
## Experiences Of a Caregiver

### Rev. Frederick A. Trunk

This is a story about the experiences of a caregiver.
He takes care of his wife, and was caregiver for another
couple who were challenged with Alzheimer's disease. The
message is, "Get help as soon as you realize
there is a challenge!"

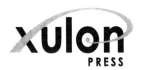
xulon
PRESS

# Table of Contents

IN LOVING MEMORY OF OUR BELOVED
GRANDDAUGHTER VICTORIA ANN LANGTON WHO
WENT TO BE WITH OUR LORD AT THE AGE OF TWENTY
THREE MONTHS BUT SPREAD MORE JOY IN EGLESTON
CHILDREN'S HOSPITAL IN ATLANTA, GEORGIA THEN MOST
PEOPLE SPREAD IN A LIFETIME

*Jesus said in Mark 10:14-15*

*Suffer the little children to come unto me, and*
*forbid them not: for of such is the kingdom of God.*

*Verily I say unto you, Whosoever shall not receive the*
*kingdom of God as a little child,*
*he shall not enter therein.*

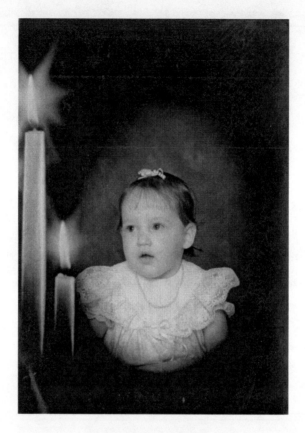

**Victoria Ann Langton**
**1990 - 1992**

*The Lord is my light and my salvation; whom shall I fear?*
*The Lord is the strength of my life; of whom*
*shall I be afraid? Psalm 27:1*

# Acknowledgments

Special thanks to the individuals and organizations listed herewith for permission to use their copyrighted material.

The Alzheimer's Association of Georgia – 800-272-3900

Santina L. Siena, M.D., Clinical Assistant Professor of Ob-Gyn, Warren Alpert Medical School, Brown University – Women & Infants Hospital, Providence, Rhode Island.

Rev. Glen Kohlhagen, Chaplain, Hospice Care Options, and Pastor of Milledgeville Presbyterian Church, Milledgeville, Georgia.

Dr. Erwin W. Lutzer, Senior Pastor, Moody Memorial Church, Chicago, Illinois.

Stephen Brown, Hawthorne, New Jersey, for the cover illustration.

Marcia Bryan, Librarian, Jefferson High School, Jefferson, Georgia. – Proof reading.

Ann Weeks Hilliard, M. Ed., National Board Certified Teacher - Editing

# Endorsements

*A*s a caregiver for my brother and mother, I can recommend this book. I have known the author for over forty five years. We still keep in touch and have talked many times about the book.

Remember your loved one is most unfortunate to have been stricken with this terrible disease. To help them you must listen to their problems or concerns and be very attentive and agree with what they are saying because you are their only outlet.

Sometimes the going may become unbearable and you think you can no longer bear the cross. Ask for God's help and He will help you carry the cross. Remember part of the prayer of St. Francis of Assisi, "it is through giving that we receive."

When it comes time for the Lord to call your loved one home you can rest in peace of mind, heart and soul that you did all that was humanly possible for them. Your comfort mean't a lot to them. As a caregiver I have two words to remember, Patience and Fortitude.

*Joseph Maltino, Caldwell, New Jersey*
*Retired Western Union Service Coordinator and Dispatcher*

As a caregiver myself with my husband Paul and sister Leona, we can recommend this book to all caregivers as well as to those who may know someone who is challenged with either dementia or Alzheimer's. I have known the author for over forty five years and was a member of an organization he founded for fellowship and to assist church musicians to improve their performance and help them with the appropriate selection of and presentation of church music. He also instructed me in the use of the church organ.

He was adept at planning and organizing whatever he put his hand to and his experience as a caregiver for his beloved wife both at home and now in a nursing facility equips him with first hand knowledge to write a book, with empathy, for caregivers.

*Myna Dumbert, Lincoln Park, New Jersey*
*Retired Bell Atlantic Telephone Company Representative*

# Preface

*A*fter my wife, Marjorie Trunk, was diagnosed with the onset of Alzheimer's disease in 2001, our lives were completely changed. Because of the effects of this terrible disease and as time goes by the changes become more challenging and life changing. Many of the things that it does affect not only for the patient, but also for the caregivers and those related to the patient, be it family or friends, will be dealt with later in the book.

I decided to write this book to help caregivers and their families know what to expect and possibly make some suggestions from my experiences to help with the situation.

Over the years I have noticed and actually come in contact with people who have family and friends with various stages of dementia and Alzheimer's. I am amazed at how much they don't know about these diseases and how overwhelmed and frustrated they can become.

It is evident that every patient is a little different but after talking with many caregivers and social workers about the disease, one can see the similarities that occur with each patient.

An interesting fact to know is that Marjorie had four sisters and one brother who also had Alzheimer's or dementia, and four of the five spent their last years in a nursing facility. These figures may change in time.

As the youngest of three brothers and six sisters, one

may assume that the disease may be hereditary. This is a personal opinion since the Alzheimer's Association does not state that nor has it been proven.

I have Aunts, Uncles and Grandparents who lived to be eighty five or more and one Aunt lived to be one hundred. None of them had any signs of Alzheimer's or dementia. A few of them had what we all call "Senior Moments." I get those at 74, but still have a sharp mind and am able to do for myself without any help from others.

I trust that the information and experiences in this book will help to aid many in their caregiving position. Although none of us wish to be in this situation our love for the individual with the challenge, enables us to serve with love, and the peace and grace that only our Lord can give us. We do our best until the very end.

I learned early on to ask for help, get involved with a support group and learn as much as I can about the disease. I thank myself for doing so.

# Chapter One

# What is Alzheimer's?

*M*emory loss in varying degrees comes first. In recent years the more common term for those who have dementia is Alzheimer's disease.

The three stages or phases of what eventually is Alzheimer's disease are all a deterioration of the brain.

Brain dysfunction is the loss of ability to reason and to remember. The brain is an immensely complex organ composed of an estimated one hundred billion nerve cells or neurons and billons more cells, called glial cells. Each neuron receives an enormous amount of information to it from thousands of other cells.

In 1906 Alois Alzheimer, a German neurologist, first described a form of cognitive impairment in humans that has come to be called Alzheimer's disease. As you will see later in this book, it all starts with some memory loss. When you start writing notes to yourself to remember things, it is starting. Also memory loss that disrupts your daily life such as forgetting recently learned information. Others include forgetting important dates and events; asking for the same information over and over; relying on memory aides or family members for things they used to handle on their own.

Some people may experience changes in their ability to develop and follow a plan or work with numbers. They may have difficulty following familiar recipes or keeping track of monthly bills. They may also have difficulty concentrating and take much longer to do things than they did before.

They may experience difficulty completing familiar tasks at home, at work or at leisure. They may have trouble driving to a familiar location or remembering rules of a favorite game.

People with Alzheimer's/dementia can lose track of time or dates, seasons and the passage of time. Sometimes they forget where they are or how they got there. In the later stages they have trouble with visual images as well as problems with words in speaking or writing.

It is very common for them to misplace things and place them in very unusual places. It is common for them to withdraw from social activities, have mood and personality changes and become confused.

Alzheimer's is not a respecter of age. It has been known that people as young as thirty has been challenged with full blown Alzheimer's. This is rather scary to think about. The percentage of those getting the disease before the age of sixty is about 0.1 percent, then it jumps to about forty seven percent after the age of eighty to eighty five.

There are as many as 5.4 million people living with the disease in the United States. This figure represents some 5.2 million people over 65 and about 200,000 people under 65 with younger-onset Alzheimer's disease.

There are some misconceptions about where Alzheimer's comes from. You may have heard that it can come from aluminum cans and cooking pots. It has also been said that artificial sweeteners such as Nutrasweet and Sweet and Low can cause the disease but that is a myth. Other myths are that it can come from flu shots and silver dental fillings.

In 2011, a survey was taken to find out what Americans think about being tested for Alzheimer's and what drugs are available to help delay or cure the disease. Nearly sixty percent of Americans said they believe there's a reliable medical test for the disease, and close to half of them believe that there is now an effective treatment to slow the progression of the disease.

Unfortunately, neither of those things is true, at least not yet. There are exciting strides toward a reliable test and drug companies vie to bring the first diagnostic tests to market. It will likely be many years before any test can predict who will get the disease, and when.

It is important to understand the disease and to understand its impact on society as well as your loved ones. Understanding the disease process is very important especially for caregivers and family members. At this time there are only theories about the causes of the disease.

It is important to know and understand the affects on the brain and how it is diagnosed and treated. The Alzheimer's Association has chapters and caregivers groups in most states. They are very willing to send out literature and books regarding the disease.

It wasn't until the early 80's that public awareness was started by groups focusing on the disease and Congressional recognition of the social and financial costs of its devastating effects, and the appropriation of more than half of the budget of the National Institute on Aging to work for a cure. As of now there is still no cure however there are a few medications that can delay the process of the disease.

# Chapter Two

# A background

*M*arjorie and I were married on June 28, 1958 in our church in Newark, New Jersey at 3:30 PM.

Her affiliation with the church came a few years earlier, when her Father, a retired minister came to the church with his family. Marjorie taught Sunday School for quite a few years before and after we were married.

I was already the Music Director/Organist having filled the position of organist since I was fifteen years of age, and then going on to be the Music Director.

After we were married, Marjorie was told that she could not have children so we proceeded to adopt.

In February of 1965, we picked up our beautiful baby girl whom we named Susan Ruth. She was the joy of our lives. Immediately we applied for a second adoption so that we would have two children about three years apart.

We, of course, are not the only couple to tell this story, but we applied for a second baby girl. Soon afterwards Marjorie started not feeling too well so we went to the doctor and he told us that he thought she was pregnant. To be sure he would take the rabbit test, which I know dates us, and if the rabbit dies, she's pregnant.

The rabbit died, and on December 30, 1967, Marjorie gave birth to a 9 pound 10 ounce baby boy that had jet black hair and looked like a three or four month old baby.

In fact, he got so much attention in the hospital nursery that it was all around the hospital, "Did you see the Trunk baby?" We named him David Frederick.

So, we have an adopted daughter and a biological son. Is there any difference many ask? No! To us they are just "both ours."

When Marjorie was planning our wedding, she told me that she never wanted to marry a minister because of all of the "challenges" that a PK (pastor's kid) had to endure. When our children were a little older, and since I had a position with a well known music company, I was able to arrange my schedule so that I could start college and work for both a bachelors degree and a masters degree.

After many years of study and hard work, I was able to get a B.M. (Bachelor of Music). After we moved to the Atlanta area, I went on to earn a M.M. (Masters of Ministry) and was ordained as a Minister of Music.

Marjorie was not disappointed in my achievements and worked with me in many of the churches where she sang in my choirs and helped in the Hand Bell choir.

In her early years she would sing trios with her sisters in their father's church and later in my church.

Over the years, I have served in nine churches for more then fifty years and still actively serve in a local church. Marjorie held down secular positions after our children were grown, and her mind was always very strong. She performed many tasks and jobs that one would think would only be done by someone who had college behind them. Although she had no college degrees she did well in the business world, kept a spotless home, and kept our children the same way.

The background that I am giving you is to show the reader that we were what one might call the "average American family." Both Marjorie and I were active not only socially, but in our faith and in the business world. Neither of us ever had any shortness of memory.

# Chapter Three

# The Years Just Prior
# to Diagnoses

*F*or her entire life up until 1998, Marjorie was physically fit. In 1958 she had an ovarian cyst removed, then in 1967 gave natural birth to our Son David, but other then that she was considered a healthy well adjusted female mother of two. In 1984, I took a position with the Rodgers Instrument Corporation in Hillsboro, Oregon as Regional Sales Manager. I was responsible for the entire Southeastern United States and the Caribbean so I was often gone during the week however Marjorie continued to maintain our rather large home in Peachtree City, Georgia and even did some volunteer work for our church and the community.

One day I was at home, and she said she didn't feel well. When I asked her what she thought was wrong, she said "Oh, I must have a virus or cold." That day I gave her cold medicine and hot soup but she seemed to throw it all up.

I was giving her aspirin during the day because she had a low fever. Nothing that I thought required the doctor let alone the hospital.

That evening when it was bed time, I went up to her with some aspirin and a warm flu medication but she didn't want it, so I said, "If you are not better tomorrow, you are going to the doctor." She agreed. At that, she got up to go to the bathroom, and just slid down to the floor and was talking irrationally.

That was it! I called 911, and within a short period of time she was in the Fayetteville Hospital, in Fayetteville, Georgia.

She was soon diagnosed with Septicemia, a life threatening blood infection.

During her first five days in the hospital, while in ICU, she suffered a severe heart attack and as soon as she was able they transferred her to Piedmont Hospital in Atlanta where they inserted stents to take care of two 95 percent blockages in her heart. This all took place in April of 1998. Marjorie did quite well after her recuperation from the ordeal, but the doctor did not want her to deal with steps, so we put our house on the market and asked her cardiologist if he felt it was wise to make a move to Florida. There we could officially retire and downsize to a more manageable home, and Marjorie would be able to completely recuperate from the illness she experienced in April.

He agreed and of course we arranged for doctors for both of us before we even made the move. So our plans to retire and do the wonder things that retired people do was now on the agenda.

We made our move to Florida and purchased a beautiful triple wide manufactured home in a retirement community in Plant City, Florida.

We had many friends all throughout the central part of Florida so we were looking forward to a lot of good times. As we anticipated, we did enjoy just about two years of wonderful traveling to places where we had not been and visiting friends we had not seen for quite some time. We got involved in church and I continued my ministry as Minister of Music, and also played the wonderful organs at two theatres in the area, namely The Tampa Theatre in Tampa, and the Lakeland Theatre in Lakeland, Florida. I was also the organist for the Plant City Cornerstone Community Center.

During these first two years Marjorie was active with me

but along about early 2001 she seemed to have a problem writing, and could not remember things such as our phone numbers, our street address and other things that may not seem important and some might say well that was just a "Senior Moment," but I got quite concerned and made arrangements for her to see a neurologist. Also during this time she had some TIAs. The medical name for this is, "transient ischemic attack" – meaning there is a temporary blockage of the blood supply to the brain, causing a temporary lack of oxygen. Usually the symptoms disappear quickly. They are sometimes referred to as a mini stroke. We both believe that having these left her with weakness in the left leg and on a number of occasions she fell. Since the house was all carpeted she never hurt herself seriously but it concerned us that she might fall outside either on the walkway or the pavement where we often took walks and walked our dog. This weakness continues to this day.

We saw the neurologist, and he gave Marjorie some writing tests and asked her questions about her daily activities, and tried his best to figure out what the problem was. He finally told us that she had the early onset of Parkinson's disease.

The doctor put her on a medication called sinimet and also referred us to a support group for Parkinson's disease and diseases that affect the motor skills.

As you will read later in this book the mid and late stages of Alzheimer's also affects motor skills. The group meetings were for more then just Parkinson's patients and their families. We did not know at this time however that Marjorie would soon be diagnosed with the early onset of Alzheimer's.

We went to quite a few of these meetings. Marjorie's condition did not get better nor did it get dramatically worse.

Sometime later during the year 2001, she went to her primary doctor because she had symptoms similar to an allergy. The doctor examined her and sent her on her way thinking she just had an allergy.

Her nose seemed to be quite swollen and I was not happy about the fact that the doctor seemed to just lightly pass it off as an allergy, something she had never had before.

I suggested we go to another doctor for a second opinion, and let me say here that you should never be hesitant or ashamed of getting a second opinion. It paid off for us and may well have saved Marjorie's life.

This second doctor immediately recognized what turned out to be a malignant tumor in her nasal passage up near where the sinuses begin.

With this finding he immediately referred her to an Ear, Nose and Throat specialist.

# Chapter Four

# Surgery, Radiation and Chemotherapy

*T*he ENT doctor immediately recognized the tumor and told us that it could be benign or malignant. We wouldn't know until the tumor was removed and biopsied. The results showed that it was a B Cell Lymphoma Cancer. Radiation and chemotherapy would be necessary to kill any of the tumor that could be left in the nose after the surgery. I want to mention here that I am not recommending any physicians or treatments as every situation is different; however, our experiences could very well be helpful to anyone who is seeking other opinions.

Marjorie was admitted to St. Joseph's Hospital in Tampa, Florida for the surgery.

It is probably the only hospital in the Tampa area that has a whole wing dedicated to cancer treatment.

Marjorie came through with flying colors and shortly after the surgery treatments were set up with an oncologist and a radiologist.

While she was hospitalized one of her examining doctors questioned her use of sinimet (Parkinson's medication). After completing his examination he told us that she did not have Parkinson's, took her off of the medication and continued treating the problems that were obvious. Again, I stress the importance of second opinions.

We were assured at this point by the oncologist that

with the proper treatment Marjorie could be cancer free and live a full and productive life. Although cancer is no longer a death sentence, Marjorie and I had never had any experience with cancer or the treatment there of, and of course we certainly didn't know what questions to ask.

Before beginning the treatments the oncologist set up thirty hypobaric treatments. These treatments were given to boost the body's immune system in preparation for the destruction that the radiation and chemotherapy cause.

For thirty business days Marjorie would go to St. Joseph's Hospital, put on a surgical gown and sit in a chamber that is especially designed to give pure oxygen to the body, thus building up the immune system. It is not painful and five to six individuals could go in the chamber at the same time.

After these treatments we were all set to start radiation and chemotherapy.

I must point out here that radiation is rough on the body even though it doesn't physically hurt. It burns the area where the tumor and any cancer remains after the surgery. Unfortunately, it also does other damage as does chemo. We were told in advance that a special mask would be made to fit Marjorie's face so that the radiation did not burn parts of her head that was not immediately adjacent to where the tumor was, or where there was no cancer. We were never told that radiation would in time rot the teeth and burn all of the saliva glands. We were quite disappointed that the doctor did not explain this in advance. By doing so, he not only would have given us a choice but we would know what to expect after the treatments.

One of the results is dry mouth which is very, very uncomfortable. After losing all of her otherwise good teeth and having to get dentures, Marjorie had a very difficult time wearing the dentures due to the dry mouth condition. Dentures need the natural moisture that is produced by our natural saliva. This moisture creates the suction that holds the dentures in place, and if taken away you have problems. This problem continues to this day. Had we known this in advance, Marjorie could have made her own choice as to whether or not she wanted the radiation treatments. Another effect of the radiation is that it damaged her inner ear and caused hearing loss. Although radiation kills cancer, it also leaves its mark depending on whatever part of the body it is focused on. Unfortunately, we would learn later that it also affected her brain.

# Chapter Five

# Starting To Notice Unusual Behavior

*A*fter Marjorie completed radiation and chemotherapy, she started to tell me things that I thought were unusual. Keep in mind that her mind had always been very sharp.

Occasionally, she would tell me that she saw her father walking around the bottom of our bed at night. I would ask whether it might be a dream and she would reply emphatically that she knew the difference between a dream and actually seeing someone. On some occasions she said that she saw other acquaintences who we knew, both living and deceased at the foot of the bed or wandering about the room.

I don't recall seeing anything in other publications or written articles on Alzheimer's that states that the individual tells stories that are almost believable, but it seems that Marjorie was doing this very early on. Most of the time I would listen to her story then I would try to help her rationalize it but believe me sometimes it was very hard to do. Early on she would tell me stories about individuals that were either on TV or on some of the DVDs that we watched, and there is no way on earth that she really knew this information. She would often say, "Well didn't you know that?" and usually a no would be sufficient, but sometimes she would want me to agree with her story and that was very difficult.

It meant I would have to lie about the situation, but I already knew from going to caregivers that you don't argue with a challenged person. You pacify them as best you can and sometimes that means changing the subject, or I would often say, "Well I'm going to look in to that and get back to you."

One story she told me and also told several of her doctors years later was about the time she fell in our carport.

This is what actually happened: A fire or emergency truck had entered our street (this was in the retirement park) and stopped just a few houses down from ours and I went out to see what might be going on. It stayed there quite a while but then left. I came back in to the house and told Marjorie what I saw and that it was probably just a false alarm. So, she went out on the steps to our carport and maybe spent a minute or so there and then came back in.

This is her story: "Why didn't you come out for me? I fell on the ground and hit my head and laid there for about ten minutes." I asked her if I could see her head where the big bump was suppose to be, and there was nothing. Also, I knew she was only out there for a matter of minutes. She went on for quite a few years telling this story and even told one of her doctor's about it so he ordered a brain scan and nothing showed up. She continued to think that her head hurt where she hit it. This story, not like others she told that only lasted for the time it took her to tell it, lasted for quite a few years.

Others evidences was that she could not remember our home phone number or my cell phone number.

One day out of the clear blue sky, she told me that a certain gentlemen had called and asked her if he had paid my fee for playing at his wedding. Marjorie told him that he had paid me and then hung up. The reality was that I had not been paid.

Fortunately, when she told me about the incident, I called the man back and told him that my wife made a mistake. He had not yet paid me for the service. This was sort of the straw that broke the camel's back and at this point I asked her to please not answer the phone as the answering service would get it.

There were several occasions when we would go shopping together and she was unable to walk around the store so I would ask her to sit on the bench near the cashier and I would get what we needed and come right back to her.

Bad idea, I would get back to the front where the bench was, and she was no longer there. Off I would go to find her and when I did, I would ask her why she left the bench and she would say, "I was wondering where you were, you were gone so long that I thought you forgot me." On another occasion she said she thought that I was killed by an automobile.

I did not over react but soon started shopping without her. I soon made arrangements for her to see the doctor and when he realized what was going on told her she shouldn't drive and she accepted his recommendation and never asked to drive again. The doctor did not tell her not to drive because she had Alzheimer's as she wasn't yet diagnosed with same. He told her that because of the dizziness and weakness from radiation treatments she should not drive.

Several friends of ours asked me, was it safe to leave her home alone since it is common for people with memory loss to wander from their home and get lost. Marjorie was just scared beyond words to go out without me, and that fear has remained to this day. Also, we had a Lasso Apso named Muffin, and as long as Muffin was by Marjorie's side, she wasn't about to go anywhere.

Now during this early period, she started to stay at home and didn't want to go to social activities, or church, or even to visit friends in the area. She also didn't want strangers or people we knew in the house.

We belonged to a large church and had many friends who would often bring cakes and nice things over, knowing that I was now a caregiver, but when I would tell her a certain individual was coming over she got very uncomfortable and would tell me not to invite them in. Once they came in she was fidgety until they left.

This unusual behavior from a lady that use to entertain my choir members two couples at a time, every Sunday night, was just simply out of character for her. I knew it was time to seek outside advice and help.

Let me say here that most people wait until the challenge becomes overwhelming before they seek help.

If you suspect that your loved one is having more then Senior Moments, then get help before you need it. I did and I thank God and myself now for doing so.

# Chapter Six

# Getting Diagnosed

O ur primary doctor recommended that I get Marjorie to a Memory Loss Clinic.

I checked out the possibilities in the Tampa area and found that there was a Memory Loss Clinic not too far from where we lived. It was part of the Memorial Hospital in Tampa, Florida.

An appointment was made and we went for our first visit to see Doctor Susan Steen, at the time she was one of the doctors who ran this Memory Loss Clinic.

Now keep in mind at this point Marjorie had a fairly obvious amount of memory loss. According to Marjorie she didn't have Alzheimer's, and also stated that her memory was fine. I'm sure that one of these days she may realize the problem, or maybe she won't. Doctor Steen took her in and examined her and tested her in various ways. She would ask her to keep in mind three words such as boat, water and house.

The doctor would then go on talking about the situation that many have with memory loss. Then she would ask Marjorie, "What were the three words I asked you to remember a few minutes ago?"

Marjorie answered, boat, then she paused quite a while, then she said water, and paused for a while, then said I can't remember the third. Doctor Steen said, "That's okay let's try a few more." So, she went on to ask Marjorie the date, our phone number, her birthdate and Social Security number.

Out of all of the questions Doctor Steen asked, Marjorie could only remember her birthday, and Social Security number, and to this day she remembers both.

The doctor showed us films from the recent brain scan she had ordered, that Marjorie had done at Memorial Hospital.

Doctor Steen explained that the white spots were the areas on the brain that are dead cells. The dead brain cells cause the dementia or Alzheimer's. Marjorie at this time, was not hearing very well and that caused her not to hear Doctor Steen say that her diagnoses was early stage Alzheimer's. In a way, I was relieved, because I don't think that anyone really wants to be told they have the disease. The doctor did put her on Aricept, but Marjorie could not take it as it made her very sick to her stomach.

I think that it is important that we now discuss and explain the various parts of the brain and what their functions are.

Since there are actually four lobes of the brain (the cerebral cortex) we will later see how the disease affects the various parts of the brain.

For now let's look at the four lobes.

There is the Frontal lobe: The functions of the frontal lobe include reasoning, planning, organizing thoughts, behavior, sexual urges, emotions, problem-solving, judging and organizing parts of speech and motor skills (movement).

The Parietal lobe: The function of the parietal lobe include information processing, movement, spatial orientation, speech, visual perception, recognition, perception of stimuli, pain and touch sensation and cognition.

The Occipital lobe: The functions of the occipital lobe include visual reception, visual-spatial processing, movement and color recognition.

The Temporal lobes: They are responsible for all auditory processing. The functions of both (left and right) temporal lobes include distinguishing and discrimination of smell and sound from other smells and sounds respectively. Between them, they control memory (right lobe) and verbal memory (left lobe), and thus, hearing, speech and memory.

In addition, there are two hemispheres of the brain, the left-brain (which controls the right side of your body) and the right-brain (which controls the left side of your body). Left brain characteristics are logic, math and scientific. Right brain characteristics are emotional, artistic, and creative.

You will see later on in this book how different parts of the brain are affected by the disease. Also, it should be noted that not everyone with the disease experiences the same symptoms in any particular order.

At this point I was introduced to the Alzheimer's Association in Tampa, Florida and was given not only some books, but a lot of information and help on what to do when.

The Alzheimer Association states that the early phase of the disease lasts about two to four years. I'm sure that this varies according to the individual. I can realistically say that for my wife it has lasted more like four to six, or even seven years.

Now, this may be because of the treatments for cancer and the early onset of her writing ability. First, they said she was starting Parkinson's disease, and then they changed it to Alzheimer's.

According to the Alzheimer's Association the things to look for in the early Phase are:

- Changes in mood and behavior.
- Changes in mood, apathy, withdrawal, but not likely thoughts of wanting to die.
- Short-term memory loss.
- Trouble finding words and/or remembering names.
- Difficulty learning new information.
- Repeats self.

- Difficulty retaining information for more than a few minutes.
- Forgets appointments, and important events.
- Confusion, getting lost while driving or in unfamiliar settings, wander aimlessly.
- Difficulty following conversations, movies, television plots.
- Difficulty with complex tasks or following directions.
- Obvious difficulty when trying to carry out activities of daily living such as planning meals, housekeeping, paying bills and balancing checkbook.
- Hoarding of items such as food or paper towels.
- Disorientation as to day, time and place, including sleep/wake problems.
- Good compensation for memory loss; may pretend to remember someone they do not recognize.
- Agitation that interferes with participation in activities.
- Decrease in social skills.
- Poor judgment and/or poor impulse control.
- Paranoia and/or suspiciousness.
- Hide things, make unwarranted accusations or blame someone else when they can't find things.
- Difficulty with self-expression.

This is a rather lengthy list for sure. Since I have experienced the start and continued worsening of the disease with my own wife, I can honestly pick out the things that pertain to her decline and almost identify which year each event happened.

As I've mentioned before, not every patient is the same, so not every patient is necessarily going to experience the same symptoms.

It should be noted that Marjorie had some of these symptoms early on and they were so obvious that even friends and acquaintances noticed the problem. Early diagnoses and early intervention by the caregiver is so helpful. My primary intention with this book is to get the word out to anyone who even vaguely suspects there is a problem, to get information and help immediately. It will not only make it easier on the caregiver, but knowing how to handle the patient is so important. There is definitely a right way and a wrong way, and the wrong way just makes the challenge worse for everyone and it certainly confuses the patient.

One of the problems that both Marjorie and I saw first hand was when we were caregivers for a couple in Peachtree City, GA. We saw some things being done by the two individuals to each other that made the problem worse. For example the husband in this case was giving his wife hard liquor so that she wouldn't complain about her back aches, and this wasn't helping at all as she would stumble around and in some instances get hurt because she either fell or bumped part of her body against a hard surface. Then the wife would cry and carry on to get his attention when what should have happened was that their children should have taken control and helped this couple in an appropriate manner. They didn't, so the task was left to others who cared. Also, had this couple been taken to the appropriate doctors they could have gotten help and most likely would have been placed in either Assisted Living or a Nursing Home Facility.

This was not done until the couple asked me if I would be their Power of Attorney and handle their affairs knowing well that they couldn't do it without help.

We went to their lawyer and got everything set up legally and Marjorie and I took care of their needs for almost three years. They both passed on shortly thereafter.

# Chapter Seven

# Early Treatment

*S*ince Doctor Steen told me that Marjorie was just in the very early stages of Alzheimer's and that there is no known cure and very few medications to treat the disease, I passed this information on to our son, David, who lived in Jefferson, Georgia and he talked with me about moving back to Georgia so that we could all be close. If Marjorie was ever to have to be placed in a nursing facility, our family wanted it to be in Georgia rather then some five hundred miles away in Florida.

At this point Marjorie showed no drastic advancement to her challenges, but I put a for sale sign in the front window of our house. In one day a couple from Michigan stopped by and said that they wanted the house, even though they had not yet seen the inside. For us, this was what I considered to be a real miracle as homes in retirement parks, especially manufactured homes don't sell quickly at all. We sold the home, called a mover, packed our things, and back to Georgia we went.

I immediately arranged for new doctors for both of us and saw all of them within a month or so of moving to Georgia.

Our wonderful doctor in Florida, Dr. Susan Steen, had provided all kinds of information as well as arranging for caregiver's groups. I had already been put on the mailing list for the Tampa Chapter of the Alzheimer's Association so I had the material and books that they send out to caregivers.

One very important thing, at least for me, is that Marjorie does not know or think that she has Alzheimer's disease. When we go out to eat or go into public places, I am never concerned about Marjorie being embarrassed because she might be confused or say the wrong thing. I always use the card that the Alzheimer's Association has provided for such situations. To this day Marjorie has never seen the card, which reads:

> My companion has memory loss, which makes it difficult for them to find the right words and understand what has been said.
>
> Thank you for your patience.

I use this card all of the time. In fact, I had it laminated so that it wouldn't get dog eared and dirty. What I usually do is give it to the person who is seating us. They in turn give it to the server and thus what might otherwise be an embarrassing situation is changed into a situation where the server addresses most or all of their questions to me. Since my wife and I have already discussed what she would like, everything runs smoothly. Thank the Lord for small blessings.

I always show Marjorie the menu and ask her what she feels like eating, and then I select something that is usually okay. Most of the time she will ask me to choose something for her that I know she will enjoy.

I use the card for doctors visits especially if it is a first time visit. I hand the card to the receptionist and ask him/her to photocopy it and place the copy in her chart where the doctor will see it before starting to examine her. I feel confident that the physician's appreciate this as well.

If an Alzheimer's patient is able to go out in public there is no reason in the world not to take them out. I try to visit

Marjorie every other day. We go to restaurants and stores at least once a week. Since she cannot walk too well, she is in a wheelchair (transport chair) that I purchased especially for the purpose of taking her out.

It is very light weight and fits easily in to the trunk of our automobile. All restaurants and public buildings are required by law to have wheelchair access and the transport chair is less bulky and easier to maneuver then a standard wheelchair.

Our son and his wife and daughter pick Marjorie up every Sunday and we all have dinner together.

# Chapter Eight

# How Marjorie took the move back in Georgia

*M*arjorie took the change rather well, and was happy to be in our new home near our granddaughter, son and wife who live in Jefferson, Georgia. I took her to see her doctors on a regular basis, but as time passed she had more and more difficulty in several areas not all of which are related to Alzheimer's.

As I look back, I feel that one of her doctors over medicated her. Keep in mind that her left leg is and was weak even when we lived in Florida, so I feel the doctor should have been more attentive to the situation. I privately mentioned this concern to one doctor in particular on several occasions.

I felt that he needed to start reducing the medication since Marjorie was having difficulty walking. She had fallen a number of times. All I was told was that the medications had to be decreased very slowly. At this point due to her weakness and dizziness, she was only going out when she had a doctor's appointment, if it was for a holiday at our son's house, or if we were eating out. The incident that put her in the hospital and then in to the nursing facility happened one Saturday when she went to use the bathroom and was unable to get off of the toilet and walk to our bed, which was only about twelve feet. I immediately called our son, and we got her to the hospital. After two days she was transferred to the nursing facility with the plan that she would receive physical therapy and most likely return home.

That never happened. After being examined by the doctors at the facility, it was determined that Marjorie was at a point where she needed continuous nursing care.

Since we were both retired and on a fixed income, we could not afford to have the in-home nursing care that was necessary at that time. She was admitted to the facility as a long term patient.

Over the next thirty to sixty days Marjorie progressed to the point where she could walk fairly well with the assistance of a walker. She was able to move around her room and for short distances in the hallways. Any other situations required the use of a standard wheelchair or transport chair. As time went on, I continued to notice a decline in her memory and a lot of confusion. She was unable to remember the names of the nurses and cnas who worked with her on a daily basis. I already knew from attending caregiver's meetings in Florida that the control of the muscles is definitely affected by Alzheimer's so it was no surprise that her incontinence was getting to be more of a problem. Although she had some good physical therapy, she had a weakness in her legs, which as I stated earlier started several years before entering the nursing facility. This continues to this day and seems to be getting worse. As you know from an earlier chapter in this book, Marjorie had permanent inner ear damage from radiation, and problems with the after effects of chemotherapy. Keeping this in mind, her balance and dizziness was and still is a problem that she has dealt with since early 2001 when she had the Lymphoma.

Before I continue, I think that it would be appropriate to write a chapter regarding the affects that Marjorie's admittance to the nursing facility has had on me as her caregiver.

# Chapter Nine

# What a Caregiver Experiences When Their Loved One Is Institutionalized

*W*hen Marjorie was admitted to the nursing facility we had been married just over fifty years. Our wedding date was June 28, 1958. I had heard from attending caregiver's meetings that when a couple is separated whether it be by death, illness, divorce, institutionalization, or for any reason, the individuals go through the same basic steps or grieving that one does when they lose a mate to death. At the time of Marjorie's admittance to the nursing facility, I hadn't given this a lot of thought. Now as I look back to September 11, 2008, I can recall my moods and experiences as if it were yesterday.

I attended a Grief Seminar at one of the Leadership Conferences that our denomination sponsored and I learned a lot.

The steps of grieving as I learned from Chaplain Glen Kohlhagen, of Hospice Care Options, Milledgeville, Georgia, are:

- Shock
- Denial
- Extreme Sadness
- Bargaining with Supreme Authority
- Depression

- Anger
- Acceptance

I know that I have experienced some of these steps, but I can't honestly say that I've experienced all of them, but may in the future.

Grief doesn't necessarily have a time frame. It is different with everyone; however, it is generally thought that it runs for three to six months in a death situation. With other grief causing traumas such as divorce, loss of a job institutionalization etc., it is known to last longer.

In some very rare cases people have been known to grieve for years. If that is the case professional help should be considered.

There are things that you can do to help yourself handle the challenge, such as:

- Be patient and realistic
- Plan ahead
- Make lists
- Prioritize!
- Be aware of your needs
- It is okay to say "no"

Also, listen to your heart, acknowledge your limits.

Talk with others. I have found that talking to others is very enlightening and helpful. When possible I talk to family members of the patients on the same unit as my wife. I am able to encourage them and talk to them about their particular situation. We often do this at the caregiver's meetings. Share as often as you can. Back to visitation.

In the very beginning I would visit the nursing facility every day. I knew from having my mother in a nursing home for eight years that the social workers and the caregiver's meeting monitors tell you that it is not a good idea for the family to visit everyday.

Doing so doesn't allow the patient to become familiar with the surroundings and the other patients on their own. Also, it is very stressful for the spouse or family member who visits every day. As I already stated, I did visit every day but soon realized that I was actually zapping myself of energy that was necessary to live my own life and also to be a good visitor when I did go.

As of November 28, 2008, I tried to visit every other day, but if I was under the weather, had appointments, or needed to take care of personal matters I did skip days.

The longer Marjorie is at the facility the more comfortable she feels and actually considers the place her home. She has made friends with many of the patients on her floor. She eats many of her meals in the day room where she fellowships with the other patients at her table of eight or ten. In the beginning it was as though my wife had already passed away since I would come home to an empty house after each visit. The empty house caused me to imagine what it would be like if she had already passed, so I would try to keep busy doing things knowing that she was not coming home. After a while, I went through a period where I felt very depressed. I told my doctor, and he put me on an antidepressant that made me so tired that I had to stop taking it. As time passed, however, I felt stressed and tight in my chest so he again put me on something that was much milder.

Since I was and still am serving as Minister of Music and Organist in a local church, I have keep busy with my music etc., and the depression period soon passed.

As for a period of anger, I really can't say that I went through that as I have a very strong faith. I don't believe that we should become angry; however, I am told that anger may come at a later date. It's okay to be angry. God made us, He knows our feelings and accepts them. I pray for the peace and grace of our Lord to help me with the situation. I can truly say He does give me the peace in my heart to accept a situation that I have no control over.

As time moved on and Marjorie was more accepting of her situation, it has helped me to accept our circumstances. As I do with everything in my life, I take it one day at a time and I pray for guidance and the ability to figure out or work out each challenge that comes my way.

I still come home to the empty house. I have accepted the fact that Marjorie is far better off where she is than she would be if I were caring for her 24/7. I often bring her home for an afternoon and even prepare some of her favorite things to eat while she is with me. This gives her a lift, but she often says that she doesn't really mind being at the facility. As much as she would like to be home, she does understand the good that she receives there. This helps me to feel better knowing that she feels this way.

Each visit is different. Some days she is more confused and wants to leave the facility. At other times she states that she hates it there. She does ask me constantly why she has to be there.

I explain as best I can that she needs the professional care that she would not get at home. Up to this point she still doesn't realize that she has Alzheimer's. I have already spoken to the person in charge of the caregiver's meetings, and suggested that we have a talk with her about Alzheimer's. I felt that it needs to be revealed to Marjorie that she does in fact have the challenge, so that we can put that problem of asking, to rest. After talking with the social worker we both came to the conclusion that we don't need to tell her that she has Alzheimer's because time will take care of her thought process and that will take care of the problem.

# Chapter Ten

# Moving from the First Phase to the Second Phase

*A*ccording to the Alzheimer's Associations comments and material, they say that the middle phase is typically the longest phase of the disease.

- Memory loss increases: short term memory becomes more impaired.
- Forget important information such as phone number, address, and family members' names.
- Ability to learn is increasingly impaired.
- Language and communication become more impaired; difficulty expressing needs and understanding others; unable to follow verbal instructions.
- Unable to discern dangerous situations.
- Difficulty with movement, eye-hand coordination, visual-spatial functioning.
- Wander or pace (Approximately 60% of persons with Alzheimer's disease tend to wander.)
- Need assistance with activities of daily living such as toileting, bathing, dressing, grooming and eating.
- Become confused, anxious, agitated, fearful.
- Poor impulse control.
- Behaviors associated with the disease usually increase.
- Inappropriate social behavior, may disrobe in public,

    curse or belch.
- Inappropriate sexual behavior or aggression.
- May become agitated at bath time, with dressing or going somewhere.
- Hide things, accusing others of taking the missing items.
- Experience delusions and/or hallucinations, becoming upset.
- "Shadow" (follow) the caregiver.

As I mentioned earlier, not every patient is the same. It is quite interesting to note that Marjorie is now about ten years from the day she was diagnosed. Many of her symptoms fall into the category of the Early Phase; however, she has symptoms from the Middle Stage as well as the Late Stage.

You can still talk with her on the phone and you'd think there wasn't a thing wrong with her. However, in her presence even for a short while, and there are many symptoms that come under all three categories that she is challenged with and is obvious to others.

As we entered the year 2011, I found that she was having more days of complete confusion then she had had before. Often even when I was there with her she would say, "Where am I?" "What am I doing here?"

I have been told by the nurses that she has many days like that.

She is also very fearful. If there is a change of nurses or cnas from those that are usually there she will tell me that strange people are all around and that she's afraid to be there.

What I do then is try to find out who is coming on the next shift that she is familiar with and when I tell her who it is, she will usually calm down and agree that everything is okay.

It's now January 3, 2012, and Marjorie is often fearful at night. She is having more days when she is completely confused. She will call me on the phone crying and saying that she doesn't know where she is. She will also say that no one will help her, and there is no one around anyway.

What I do is tell her to let me talk to the nurse on duty and she and I discuss it and she will either help Marjorie herself or call the Social Worker whose office is on the same floor as her room. Soon they have her calmed down and every thing is okay.

I can say that now she is asking me what to do about situations such as getting her hair done, going to Bingo, wearing her dentures as well as other things and when I tell her I want her to do certain things, she usually does what I ask. I am finding too that she asks me things such as, "Should I put my pajamas on now?" This tells me that she is not thinking for herself.

So you see how some of these challenges and/or symptoms that we have listed may come on very slowly, and yet with some patients they come all at once.

# Chapter Eleven

# Moving into the Late Phase

*L*et's talk first about the suggested overview given out by the Alzheimer's Association. They state that late phase usually lasts one to two years.

- Memory loss is severe.
- Will not recognize the caregiver.
- May not recognize self in mirror.
- Nutrition becomes a problem.
- May not remember how to eat.
- May have problems with swallowing; may choke.
- Experience weight loss.
- Difficulty walking or become bedridden.
- Incontinent of bladder and/or bowels.
- Great difficulty communicating; vocabulary may be limited to only a couple of words.
- Typically a decrease in the behaviors associated with the disease; less agitation and less combative behavior.
- Increased medical problems.
- Body is more susceptible to infections such as pneumonia, etc.
- Body begins to shut down, as the brain is no longer able to tell organs how to function.

As time goes by, Marjorie's memory loss has become

quite severe. Her confusion is getting much worse, and she is expressing anger over little things.

She is allowed to use the nurse's station phone to call me at home or on my cell phone. She usually calls me on the days that I do not visit. Since her confusion is much worse then it was, she will call me and tell me that everything there at the nursing facility is messed up, and no one knows what they are doing. She will also tell me about an incident that I will later find out never happened.

At this time she was getting her shower on Tuesday and Friday in the afternoon usually about 3:30 or 4:00 PM. She called me one day and said that she is all mixed up because they didn't give her a shower on Friday (it was Saturday) and no one knows why or when they are going to give her the shower.

I got the attending nurse on the phone and she told me that the record book showed that she had a shower on Friday, but Marjorie insisted that she didn't and she wouldn't give up on the idea until something was done.

Believe me when I say these nurses and cnas are all angels sent to us by our Lord. They have to go through all kinds of drama day in and day out, and I see first hand what even the mildest patient requires as far as their necessary care and attention goes.

So, I asked the nurse if she could have one of the cnas give her a shower even if she had one the day before because Marjorie's confusion over the situation will continue until such time as they do. The nurse was very cooperative and said that she would have one of the cnas give her the shower.

Usually once something like this is taken care of, Marjorie will settle down and most likely forget that it ever happened.

Now I'm not saying that every time my wife is confused or upset over something that the nurses or cnas have to jump at her command or even as in this case give her a shower just to settle her down, what I am saying is that often the extra little attention or whatever can really put the patient at ease, is not a problem with the staff.

Marjorie has been a patient at Northridge Nursing Facility now for over three and a half years and I can say without hesitation that the staff goes out of their way for the patients.

I have seen situations where the patient makes it impossible for the nurses to do their job, and in the case of Marjorie there have been times when she emphatically refuses to take her medications, and all the nurse can do is try and of course they have to report these incidences to her doctor. Dealing with an Alzheimer's patient can be monumental.

Our son went to pick her up to take her to his house one Sunday so that we could all have dinner together and when he got there she didn't know who he was. Again, ignoring this and doing little things to change the patients mind, usually takes care of the problem. This may not be so in the future. We sent her sister who lives in New Jersey a nice corsage to wear to her eighty fifth birthday celebration with other members of the family and I explained all of this to her on the Friday before the affair. On Saturday, she said to me, "Did you get a phone call?" So I of course said from whom as I did not know who she was talking or thinking about. She said, "The one you sent flowers to!" She couldn't think of her sister's name.

I am told by the nursing home staff that there are days that she simply is so confused about where she is that she starts to cry and tells the staff she's afraid. Then she will call me all upset and crying and wanting me to pick her up immediately and take her home. She will call early in the morning or in the early evening and want to be taken home but as we all know we can't do this and it is very stressful as well as upsetting to any caregiver.

In time, she may forget that she can make phone calls but in the mean time I deal with it and do as best I can to calm her down either by getting the nurse or cna involved.

# Chapter Twelve

# What Can You Do to Help the Patient?

*T*here are so many little things that you can do for people that either have the challenge of dementia and/or Alzheimer's disease or maybe they have something else. I could probably cover many, many pages just listing them. I am referring to people who are at home or in a nursing facility.

I am fortunate to have some ladies from our church who are always doing nice things for my wife. For example: A lovely person named Sandra and her daughter Alicia took Marjorie a lovely bouquet of flowers when I was hospitalized for eight days. Keep in mind that I always tried to visit there every other day. This made her very happy and much to my surprise she remembered Alicia's name.

These same ladies as well as our friends Barbara, and J.J. are always sending nice cards and notes. Now keep in mind, Marjorie really doesn't know these individuals as she was already challenged before I was hired at the church.

Now, you might think, well they are doing that because of me, but I know for a fact that they do it for others and I say God bless them. If everyone would give one hour of their time per year, do you realize how much cheer could be spread.

Don't be afraid to approach a challenged person as we don't really know what they do or don't understand. A cheerful hello and touch on the hand or arm can do a lot of good.

I take pieces of wrapped hard candy in my pocket and I give it to the patients that I know can have it. They smile ear to ear and always say "Thank you, Mr. Trunk." One cute lady calls me "The Reverend."

As an Ordained Minister I started a program of serving the Sacrament of Holy Communion to those that understand what we are doing. Now keep in mind any venture like this should be done only in conjunction with the Administrator or Activities Director of an institution. However, there are little things that you can do that don't require organization or special permission.

Call a facility in your area and ask what you can do to just make someone happy.

Take your church youth group to a facility in your area and have them pass out homemade (or store bought) cards with pictures and inspirational sayings on them.

Have them sing a song for the patients. Often the patients will join in.

Your lady's groups can knit lap blankets and pass them out. At Christmas time you can make up little bags with goodies and a greeting card. Really there is no end to the things that we can and should do.

Now let me tell you about our Granddaughter Victoria for whom this book is dedicated. She went to be with the Lord at the age of twenty three months. When she was nine months old, she was diagnosed with AML Leukemia and spent most of the rest of her life in Egleston Children's Hospital in Atlanta, Georgia. She was walking on her own pretty much at a year old and she would go up and down the lengthy halls there at the hospital hanging on to her intravenous pole and she would go to each doorway of the patients rooms, stick her little head in and with a smile on her face say "Hi." Her vocabulary was of course very limited but she knew the word hi and used it every day to almost every one. It made the patients who were all under eighteen years of age look forward to her almost daily visits.

Her obituary stated that little Victoria spread more happiness in her short life time then most of us do in a lifetime. This shows that it only takes a word or two to spread joy or happiness especially when dealing with those who are challenged. Victoria met a need that these dear sick children needed, and you can do the same whether they are young or old.

Think about going to a children's hospital and just go around passing out little treats, or to a nursing facility where I am sorry to say that some of the patients never get a visitor.

# Chapter Thirteen

# Should We Prepare for the Death of our Loved One?

*M*y answer to this is most definitely yes. It is much easier to handle the situation of death if prearrangements are made. All funeral homes and cemeteries can make prearrangements and believe me, it makes those final few days so much easier to handle.

I have made prearrangements for my wife and myself both at the mortuary and the cemetery.

As a Minister myself I have seen and experienced many different kinds of reactions to death. My own mother passed away very unexpectedly even though she was in a nursing home, but I knew in advance what her wishes were and where she stood as far as her faith (spiritual condition).

Just recently I read a wonderful book called *One Minute After We Die,* by Dr. Erwin W. Lutzer, Senior Pastor at Moody Memorial Church in Chicago. This book is so wonderful and insightful that I am giving them to my friends and others who are interested in knowing what happens when we die.

If you can still communicate well with your challenged loved one it would serve you and your loved one well to read it.

I do believe that we see our Savior as soon as we die. An example of this is my own Granddaughter Victoria. As I told you she had AML Leukemia and we knew from the beginning that this is usually not curable. We were also told by one of the nurses that wanted us to know what to expect, that usually when death comes it is not pretty.

The patient usually bleeds from the mouth, nose and eyes. The morning that the family was all called in to the hospital (the doctors and nurses can usually tell when the end is near) my wife, our daughter, and son-in-law took turns holding Victoria in their lap, rocking her very gently.

My wife would sing quietly in her ear "Jesus Loves Me This I Know" and she would just lie there very quietly. Then while my daughter held her, all of a sudden she let out a rather loud "Ooooh," and passed. We know that when she did that then she saw Jesus and was in His loving arms.

For all of us that was a miracle in itself. We didn't have to experience what the nurses told us that the end would be like.

It reminds me of the scripture on the memorial page where Jesus said to those around Him "Suffer the little children to come unto me."

We know she's in heaven because one minute after she died, she was with the Lord.

# Chapter Fourteen

# Interviews With Other Caregivers

*A*s I was writing the chapter on "What We Can Do To Help the Patient." I was thinking that I should interview other caregivers and see just what their comments and concerns were.

So this chapter will be made up entirely of such interviews.

The first one is very close to home as the expression goes since the challenged one is Marjorie's best friend since they were in high school, so they have been close friends for well over sixty years.

Even though Emma and Richard eventually moved to the west coast, we have remained close friends visiting one another whenever possible and staying in touch via snail mail, e-mail and telephone.

We will only use first names in these interviews.

### Interview with Richard

In this interview with Richard, the husband is the caregiver. It's interesting to note here that when I was talking with one of the top individuals at the Alzheimer's Association National Headquarters in Chicago, Illinois, I was told that most books on the subject are written by female caregivers, so Richard (the caregiver in this interview) and I may be in the minority when it comes to caregiving. Maybe too this will help some of the male caregivers as they deal with their challenged mate or friend.

I was quite surprised when I realized that Emma was starting to experience memory loss and confusion. I noticed this some time back and did mention it to Richard, and he agreed.

In our interview I asked him when he first realized that Emma was challenged and his answer was about a year ago. What surprised me was how quickly she went from not challenged to very challenged. Earlier in this book I mentioned at least once and maybe more that every situation is different.

Some of Emma's experiences are much further in to the challenge then Marjorie, and she was diagnosed ten or so years ago.

I asked Richard if Emma realizes that she has a challenge, and Richard said yes. Emma still lives at home with Richard but they are planning to sell their house in Arizona and move to California near their only daughter and this will be a tremendous help to Richard. Also, should Emma need to have inpatient care at a facility, they will all be in the same area. This is why Marjorie and I moved back to Georgia after retiring and moving to Florida.

I asked Richard what his primary (not his first) concerns were for Emma, and he said eating properly and taking prescribed medications.

Richard stated that he has never attended a caregivers meeting.

Richard said that his first concern is, what would happen to my wife if I should pass on before her, or if I became disabled. To prepare for this he said that he has already given their daughter the "Power of Attorney" and he is working on a "Living Will." This is something everyone should consider.

Unfortunately, Emma is already to the phase where

she forgets her husband's name and who he is. She was always close with her brothers, and often calls Richard by her deceased brother's names. She is confused most of the time and if her digital watch says 9:15 a.m., and the clock by the bed says 9:17 a.m. she is confused and complains that she can never tell what time it is.

Richard states that he can no longer tell Emma ahead of time that they have an appointment. She will get dressed and ready to go with her purse in hand and the appointment may be hours away.

I am fortunate that Marjorie still knows me and our family members.

I pray for Richard daily as I can understand what he is going through. He doesn't get a break from the challenge. I encourage him to get some help to give himself a little time alone.

### Interview with Linda

This interview is very close to home. Linda is Marjorie's niece. The challenged one was Marjorie's brother, Lee. At the age of 92 Lee had a heart attack and several stents were inserted to take care of the blockages.

Just prior to this Linda states that she and her sisters felt that he was starting to have some memory loss. At age 95, his wife passed away and Linda was his caregiver until he went in to a nursing facility.

While he was at home a professional was brought in the home to take care of his needs during the day. At night another professional was brought in since he would be up during the night a good part of the time.

After a time the people brought in to care for Lee stated they could no longer handle him so arrangements were made for him to be placed in a nursing facility. Linda and her sister's Gloria and Geri visited him regularily.

Lee did not realize he was challenged but often did not know the people that were visiting him. When they told him who they were, he would often remember.

One day when Gloria went to visit Lee, there were fire engines and emergency vehicles outside the facility and when she got inside, found out that her father had pulled the fire alarm.

Lee passed away three months shy of his ninety ninth birthday. While living in the nursing home Lee's daughters were told about caregiver's meetings but they did not attend any since they felt it was pointless at that late time in the patient's life.

Linda encourages anyone who feels that their loved one shows even the slightest symptoms of the disease, to get help immediately.

### Interview with Karen

Karen and her family are the full time caregivers for Margie, Karen's mother who is now 80. Margie was living in an assisted living facility for about five years. About four years ago Karen noticed that she was having memory loss. About two years in to her stay at the facility Karen states that her mother started having hallucinations and was frightened at night.

Karen's sister is a nurse and trained Karen in caregiving and what is necessary to take care of a person with Alzheimer's. Since Karen's family totals five individuals and her husband David works from home four days of the week, Karen decided to bring her mother home to live with them and care for her. Karen does many innovative things to make Margie's care what it should be. One thing they decided to do since Margie is on twenty seven medications, they made a chart and placed it on the refrigerator. Whoever is in charge at a given time checks the chart and sees to it that the proper medication is given at the proper time.

Since Karen use to volunteer at the assisted living facility she has had experience working with Alzheimer patients. At times Margie does not know Karen and David but they know how to handle that and all turns out well. Margie has a one hundred pound Labrador Retreiver that she loves, and it gives her much comfort and joy. People with Alzheimer's usually take to pets very well, especially to dogs and cats.

I asked Karen if she had any concerns at this time and she said that at this time her only concern was the possibility that Margie's oxygen might come off while she is sleeping.

Karen mentioned that most people shy away from their situation with the challenged one. Some of the phases of the disease are frightening but you need to provide an anchor for yourself. Remember get help. Talk about the situation. There are plenty of people out there who are willing to help. A little help from a lot of people goes a long way.

# Chapter Fifteen

# Closing Thoughts

*T*he main purpose for this book is to help caregivers and individuals who know caregivers who are looking for answers to the many and varied questions that can come up when a loved one or friend is challenged. For this reason I am concluding this book at this time even though Marjorie is still residing at Northridge and is doing okay physically, she is becoming more challenged mentally as time goes by. It is possible that I may add to this book at a later date, or even write a second edition.

We live in the rolling hills of Northeast Georgia where from early Spring to late Fall the country side is just filled with beautiful flowers of all kinds. As I drive the back roads between our home and Northridge Nursing Facility it is primarily farm country. Wild flowers, as well as many flowers and flowering trees that are planted by individuals, are all along the fields and roadside. Because of this I felt I wanted to add my writing, "The Flower." We need to remember that God has planted us where we are for a reason. The reasons are many and also varied but we all need to consider our place in life and ask our Lord to show us what He wants us to do where we are planted. Some time back when one of our friends was challenged with a nonrelated condition such as Alzheimer's, I was lead to write a scenario about how we all need our supreme being, God, in our hearts and lives.

### The Flower

*We can see God even in a flower.*
*The pedals surround the face or eye of*
*the flower just as God's love surrounds us.*
*The face or eye of the flower reminds us that*
*"His Eye is on the Sparrow" so even*
*more so, His eye is on us in times of trouble*
*and sorrow.*
*The stem of the flower supports the head*
*of the flower holding it upright toward heaven*
*and likewise our Lord is our foundation*
*holding us up and sustaining*
*us through every phase of our lives.*
*The leaves, which often encompass the stem*
*and the face of the flower reminds us*
*that no matter what, our Lord*
*encompasses us with His, love, concern*
*strength, comfort and every other*
*supportive thing that we can name.*
**Savor the beauty of the flower and seek the Savior.**

As stated in an earlier chapter Marjorie and I have always had a strong faith and I encourage everyone to hold on to their faith, cherish the Savior and your family and friends. In our case, we have so many friends that do wonderful things not only for Marjorie but also for me. Little things can mean a lot when a caregiver needs help or the challenged person is not doing so well.

Our church family is a tremendous support in many, many ways. Don't hesitate to reach out and ask for help. Sometimes people are just waiting to be asked or told what the need is. They often hold back until you ask because they don't want to be intrusive. There are also many organizations out there that can be of help. Again, you need to ask.

You can feel free to e-mail me if you have any comments or questions regarding what I have written.

FrederickAT263@aol.com

<u>NOTES</u>

CPSIA information can be obtained at www.ICGtesting.com
Printed in the USA
BVOW07s0205251013

334598BV00008B/52/P